THE LOW FODMAP DIET FOR BEGINNERS

Guide yourself toward improving Digestive health by exploring delicious and healthy recipes to relieve digestive disorder,Allowing you to play an active role in your well-being.

Table of contents

Introduction

The Low FODMAP Diet is a dietary approach designed to alleviate symptoms associated with irritable bowel syndrome (IBS) and other functional gastrointestinal disorders. FODMAPs, which stands for Fermentable Oligosaccharides, Disaccharides, Monosaccharides, and Polyols, are certain types of carbohydrates that can trigger digestive discomfort in some individuals.

This diet involves restricting the intake of specific FODMAP-containing foods for a period, followed by a systematic reintroduction phase to identify individual tolerance levels. The primary goal is to reduce the fermentation of these carbohydrates in the gut, which can lead to symptoms such as bloating, gas, abdominal pain, and altered bowel habits.

For beginners, understanding the categories of high and low FODMAP foods is crucial. High FODMAP foods include certain fruits, vegetables, grains, dairy products, and sweeteners, while low FODMAP alternatives are generally better tolerated. It's essential to work with a healthcare professional or a registered dietitian when embarking on the Low FODMAP Diet, as they can provide personalized guidance and ensure nutritional adequacy during the elimination and reintroduction phases.

This diet is not a one-size-fits-all solution, and individual responses to specific FODMAPs vary. Therefore, a well-structured introduction to the Low FODMAP Diet involves education, support, and careful guidance to help individuals navigate the complexities of the diet and identify trigger foods for their unique digestive sensitivities.

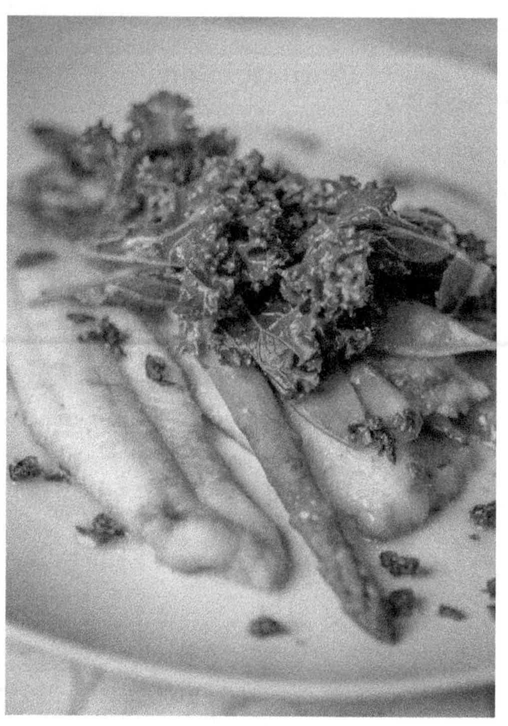

CHAPTER ONE

UNDERSTANDING FOOD MAP

Understanding FODMAPs involves identifying and managing these compounds in the diet to alleviate symptoms like bloating and abdominal discomfort, especially for those with irritable bowel syndrome (IBS).

WHAT IS FODMAP

Fermentable Oligosaccharides, Disaccharides, Monosaccharides, and Polyols are a class of sugar alcohols and short-chain carbohydrates that go by the acronym FODMAPs.

A low FODMAP diet is designed to reduce the intake of these compounds, as they can trigger digestive symptoms in some individuals. This dietary approach aims to alleviate symptoms associated with irritable bowel syndrome (IBS) and other functional gastrointestinal disorders. By limiting the consumption of foods rich in FODMAPs, individuals may experience relief from bloating, gas, and abdominal discomfort. The low FODMAP diet involves careful selection of foods to manage these fermentable substances and can be an effective strategy for improving digestive well-being in susceptible individuals.

FERMENTABLE OLIGOSACCHARIDES, DISACCHARIDES, MONOSACCHARIDES, and POLYOLS

Fermentable Oligosaccharides, Disaccharides, Monosaccharides, and Polyols (FODMAPs) refer to specific types of carbohydrates that are known to cause digestive discomfort in some individuals, particularly those with irritable bowel syndrome (IBS). Let's break down each component:

1. Fermentable: These carbohydrates are easily fermented by bacteria in the gut, leading to the production of gases such as carbon dioxide, methane, and hydrogen. This fermentation process can cause bloating, gas, and other gastrointestinal symptoms.

2. Oligosaccharides: These are carbohydrates composed of a few sugar molecules linked together. The main types of oligosaccharides in FODMAPs are fructans and galacto-oligosaccharides (GOS). Common sources include wheat, onions, garlic, and certain legumes.

3. Disaccharides: Two sugar molecules combine to form these types of carbohydrates. . Lactose, a type of disaccharide found in milk and dairy products, is a common Fodmap.Consuming foods high in lactose might cause digestive problems for those who are lactose intolerant.

4. Monosaccharides: These are single sugar molecules. The monosaccharide in FODMAPs is fructose, which is naturally present in fruits and some vegetables. Some people may experience symptoms due to an impaired ability to absorb excess fructose.

5. Polyols: Also known as sugar alcohols, polyols are sugar substitutes that can be found naturally in certain fruits and vegetables or added to processed foods. Examples of polyols in FODMAPs include sorbitol, mannitol, and xylitol. They may contribute to symptoms like bloating and diarrhea and have a laxative impact.

COMMON SOURCES OF FODMAP IN EVERYDAY FOODS.

Common sources of FODMAPs (fermentable oligosaccharides, disaccharides, monosaccharides, and polyols) in everyday foods include:

1. Oligosaccharides:
   - Wheat products (bread, pasta)
   - Onions
   - Garlic
   - Legumes (beans, lentils)
2. Disaccharides:
   - Dairy products (milk, yogurt, cheese)
   - Some fruits (apples, cherries, peaches)
   - Sweeteners containing lactose (some processed foods)
3. Monosaccharides:
   - High-fructose fruits (apples, pears, watermelon)
   - Honey
   - Agave nectar
4. Polyols:
   - Certain fruits (avocado, blackberries, cherries)
   - Artificial sweeteners (sorbitol, mannitol, xylitol)
   - Some vegetables (cauliflower, mushrooms)

Understanding and managing FODMAP intake can be crucial for individuals with irritable bowel syndrome (IBS) or other gastrointestinal sensitivities.

HOW FODMAP CAN TRIGGER DIGESTIVE SYMPTOMS.

FODMAPs, which stands for Fermentable Oligosaccharides, Disaccharides, Monosaccharides, and Polyols, are a group of short-chain carbohydrates found in various foods. These compounds can trigger digestive symptoms in susceptible individuals due to their fermentability and osmotic properties.

1. Fermentation: FODMAPs are rapidly fermented by bacteria in the gut. Gases including carbon dioxide, methane, and hydrogen are created during this process. This fermentation can lead to bloating, abdominal distension, and flatulence.
2. Osmotic Effects: FODMAPs have osmotic properties, meaning they draw water into the intestinal tract. This increased water content in the gut can result in diarrhea or loose stools. The osmotic effects may also contribute to abdominal pain and discomfort.
3. Individual Variability: People vary in their ability to digest and absorb FODMAPs. Individuals with irritable bowel syndrome (IBS) or other functional gastrointestinal disorders may be more sensitive to the effects of FODMAPs, experiencing symptoms like abdominal pain, cramping, and altered bowel habits.
4. Poor Absorption: Some individuals lack the enzymes needed to break down certain FODMAPs in the small intestine. For instance, lactose intolerance is a common condition where the enzyme lactase, responsible for breaking down lactose, is deficient. This can lead to digestive symptoms such as gas, bloating, and diarrhea after consuming dairy products.
5. Increased Gas Production: The fermentation of FODMAPs produces gases in the colon, contributing to symptoms like bloating and flatulence. In individuals with a heightened sensitivity to gas distension, even small amounts of gas can lead to discomfort.
6. Alteration of Gut Microbiota: FODMAPs can influence the composition of the gut microbiota. Changes in the balance of gut bacteria may contribute to gastrointestinal symptoms. Certain bacterial species thrive on FODMAPs, and an overgrowth of these bacteria may exacerbate digestive issues.
7. Interaction with Nervous System: FODMAPs can interact with the gut-brain axis, influencing the communication between the gut and the central nervous system. This interaction may contribute to symptoms such as abdominal pain, bloating, and changes in bowel habits.

It's important to note that the impact of FODMAPs on digestive symptoms can vary widely between individuals. While a low-FODMAP diet may be beneficial for some with gastrointestinal issues, it's crucial to consult with a healthcare professional or a registered dietitian to ensure proper nutritional intake and personalized management.

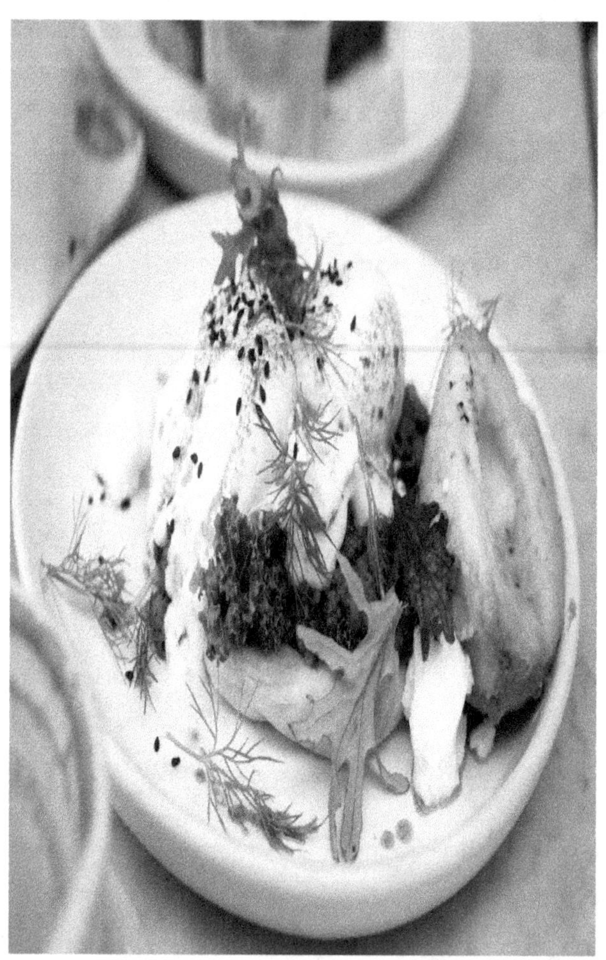

CHAPTER 2

BENEFITS OF THE LOW FOODMAP DIET

1. Symptom Reduction: The primary goal of the Low FODMAP diet is to alleviate symptoms associated with IBS, such as bloating, gas, abdominal pain, and irregular bowel movements.
2. Individualized Approach: It involves a personalized approach, as individuals can identify specific high-FODMAP foods that trigger their symptoms and customize their diet accordingly.
3. Scientifically Supported: The diet is backed by scientific research, with several studies showing its effectiveness in reducing IBS symptoms.
4. Improved Digestive Comfort: By avoiding high-FODMAP foods, individuals may experience improved digestive comfort, leading to a better quality of life.
5. Dietary Diversity: Although the elimination phase restricts certain foods, the diet encourages the reintroduction of low-FODMAP foods, promoting a more balanced and diverse diet in the long run.
6. Enhanced Nutrient Absorption: Some individuals with IBS may have difficulty absorbing certain nutrients. The Low FODMAP diet, when followed with guidance, can help ensure adequate nutrient intake.
7. Psychological Well-being: The alleviation of digestive symptoms can positively impact mental health, reducing anxiety and stress related to gastrointestinal issues.
8. Increased Energy Levels: Improved digestion and nutrient absorption may lead to increased energy levels and a general sense of well-being.
9. Better Sleep Quality: Relief from gastrointestinal discomfort can contribute to better sleep quality, as digestive issues often disrupt sleep patterns.
10. Empowerment and Control: The diet empowers individuals to take control of their symptoms and make informed choices about their diet based on their unique sensitivities.
11. Long-term Management: For those with chronic digestive issues, the Low FODMAP diet can serve as a long-term management strategy, allowing individuals to enjoy a wide variety of foods while minimizing symptom flare-ups.

IMPROVEMENTS IN OVERALL GUT HEALTH

Improving overall gut health involves fostering a balanced and diverse microbiome, which plays a crucial role in digestion, immunity, and overall well-being. Dietary choices significantly impact gut health, and incorporating fiber-rich foods like fruits, vegetables, and whole grains promotes the growth of beneficial bacteria.

Probiotics, found in fermented foods such as yogurt, kefir, and sauerkraut, can introduce beneficial bacteria to the gut. Prebiotics, on the other hand, are non-digestible fibers that nourish existing beneficial bacteria, and sources include garlic, onions, and bananas. A combination of pre- and probiotics can enhance microbial diversity.

Regular physical activity has been linked to a healthier gut microbiome, promoting the growth of diverse bacterial species. Additionally, managing stress through practices like meditation or yoga can positively impact gut health, as stress can alter the gut microbiota composition.

Adequate hydration supports digestion and helps maintain the mucosal lining of the intestines. Limiting the intake of processed foods, artificial sweeteners, and antibiotics can also contribute to a healthier gut, as these factors may negatively affect the balance of gut bacteria.

Furthermore, understanding individual responses to certain foods through elimination diets or food sensitivity testing can aid in identifying and avoiding potential triggers that may disrupt gut health. Maintaining a regular eating schedule and avoiding excessive use of antibiotics, unless prescribed by a healthcare professional, are further strategies for sustaining a healthy gut.

Overall, a holistic approach, encompassing dietary choices, physical activity, stress management, and mindful lifestyle habits, is key to fostering and maintaining optimal gut health.

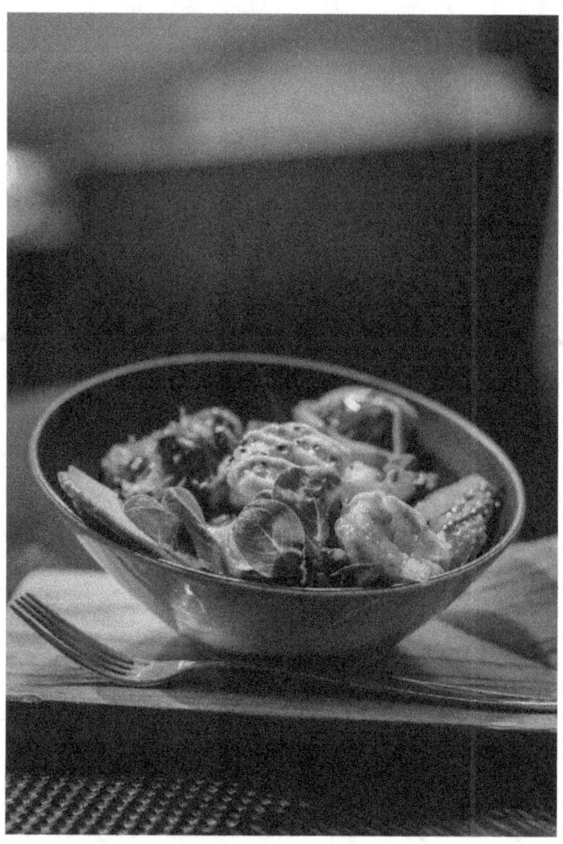

CHAPTER 3

GETTING STARTED

Starting a low FODMAP diet involves understanding and avoiding certain types of fermentable carbohydrates that can trigger digestive symptoms. Begin by researching foods high in FODMAPs and those that are safe to eat. Consider consulting a registered dietitian experienced in FODMAPs for personalized guidance. Keep a food diary to track your symptoms and gradually reintroduce FODMAPs to identify specific triggers.

PREPARING MENTALLY FOR THE DIET.

Preparing mentally for a diet can be challenging, especially if you have a history of digestive issues or food intolerances. To mentally prepare for a low FODMAP diet, you may want to consider the following tips:

- **Establish realistic expectations.** A low FODMAP diet is not a quick fix or a permanent solution. It is a temporary eating plan that helps you identify which foods cause you problems and which foods you can tolerate. You will need to follow the diet for two to six weeks, then gradually reintroduce high FODMAP foods one by one to see how they affect you. The goal is to find a balance between symptom relief and nutritional adequacy.

- **Make a commitment.** A low FODMAP diet can be restrictive and difficult to follow, especially if you eat out, travel, or have a busy lifestyle. You will need to plan ahead, read food labels, cook your own meals, and avoid certain foods and ingredients. You will also need to monitor your symptoms and keep a food diary to track your progress. To succeed, you will need to be motivated and dedicated to making a change in your eating habits.

- **Hone your inner motivation.** Ask yourself why you want to follow a low FODMAP diet. What are your goals and how will they benefit you? How will you feel when you achieve them? How will you cope with challenges and setbacks? Having a clear vision of your desired outcome and a positive attitude can help you stay focused and motivated throughout the process.

- **Key into your body's signals.** A low FODMAP diet can help you become more aware of your body's reactions to different foods. You will learn to listen to your hunger and fullness cues, as well as your symptoms and sensations. You will also learn to distinguish between physical and emotional hunger, and to avoid using food as a reward or a coping mechanism. By tuning into your body's signals, you can make more mindful and healthy food choices.

- **Be accountable.**Having a solid support network can have a significant impact on your achievement. You may want to share your goals and plans with your family, friends, doctor, dietitian, or therapist. They can provide you with emotional support, practical advice, and encouragement. You can also join online or offline groups or communities of people who follow a low FODMAP diet. You can exchange recipes, tips, experiences, and challenges with others who understand what you are going through.

- **Create a meal plan that fits your lifestyle.**A diet low in FODMAPs doesn't have to be tasteless or monotonous. There are many foods that you can enjoy, and many ways to prepare them. You can find low FODMAP recipes online or in books, or you can adapt your favorite dishes by substituting or omitting high FODMAP ingredients. You can also use spices, herbs, oils, vinegars, and sauces to add flavor and variety to your meals. You may want to plan your meals and snacks ahead of time, and stock up on low FODMAP staples and snacks. This way, you can avoid being caught off guard by hunger or cravings, and have more control over what you eat.

- **Rethink exercise.** Exercise is an important part of a healthy lifestyle, and it can also help you manage your digestive symptoms. Exercise can improve your mood, reduce stress, enhance blood flow, and stimulate bowel movements. However, some types of exercise can also worsen your symptoms, especially if you do them on an empty or full stomach, or if you are dehydrated. You may want to experiment with different types of exercise, such as walking, swimming, yoga, or pilates, and find what works best for you. You may also want to adjust the intensity, duration, frequency, and timing of your exercise according to your symptoms and tolerance·

- **Remember to be patient.** A low FODMAP diet can be a life-changing experience, but it can also be a challenging one. You may not see immediate results, or you may experience ups and downs along the way. You may also face difficulties in following the diet, such as social pressure, temptation, boredom, or frustration. Be gentle with yourself if you make errors or experience failures. Learn from them and move on. Remember that you are doing this for yourself, and that you are not alone. Celebrate your achievements, no matter how small, and reward yourself with non-food treats. Above all, never forget that you are valuable.

CLEANING OUT THE PANTRY AND FRIDGE.

Cleaning out the pantry and fridge is a task that can help you maintain a healthy and organized kitchen. Here are some steps to follow:

1. **Gather the supplies.** You will need a trash bag, a recycling bin, a compost bin, a damp cloth, a dry cloth, a disinfectant spray, and some storage containers or labels if needed.
2. **Empty the pantry and fridge.** Take out everything from your pantry and fridge and place them on a large table or counter. Your ability to recognize what you have and need to get rid of will improve as a result.

3. **Sort and discard**. Go through each item and check the expiration date, the condition, and the usefulness. Toss anything that is expired, spoiled, moldy, stale, or unwanted into the trash, recycling, or compost bin. You can also donate any unopened and non-perishable items to a food bank or a shelter.
4. **Clean the shelves and drawers**. Wipe down the inside of your pantry and fridge with a damp cloth and a disinfectant spray. Make sure to reach the corners and the back of the shelves and drawers. Dry them with a dry cloth and let them air out for a few minutes.
5. **Organize and restock**. Put back the items that you want to keep in your pantry and fridge. You can use storage containers, bins, baskets, jars, or labels to group similar items together and make them easier to find. You can also arrange them by frequency of use, type, or expiration date. For example, you can put the most used items in the front, the grains and cereals in one bin, the spices and sauces in another, and the dairy and meat products in the coldest part of the fridge. Make sure to leave some space between the items for air circulation and visibility.

By following these steps, you can clean out your pantry and fridge in a comprehensive and efficient way. And enjoy the benefits of having a cleaner, healthier meal and more organized kitchen.

Certainly! Creating a Low FODMAP meal plan involves selecting foods low in fermentable carbohydrates. Start with protein sources like chicken, turkey, or fish. Incorporate low FODMAP vegetables such as carrots, spinach, and bell peppers. Use gluten-free grains like rice or quinoa. Include lactose-free dairy or alternatives.

For a shopping list:

1. Proteins: Chicken, turkey, fish.

2. Low FODMAP veggies: Carrots, spinach, bell peppers.

3. Gluten-free grains: Rice, quinoa.

4. Lactose-free dairy or alternatives: lactose-free milk, lactose-free yogurt.

5. Fruits: Limited to low FODMAP options like berries or bananas.

6. Condiments: Check for garlic and onion-free options.

Never forget to seek individualized counsel from a registered dietician.

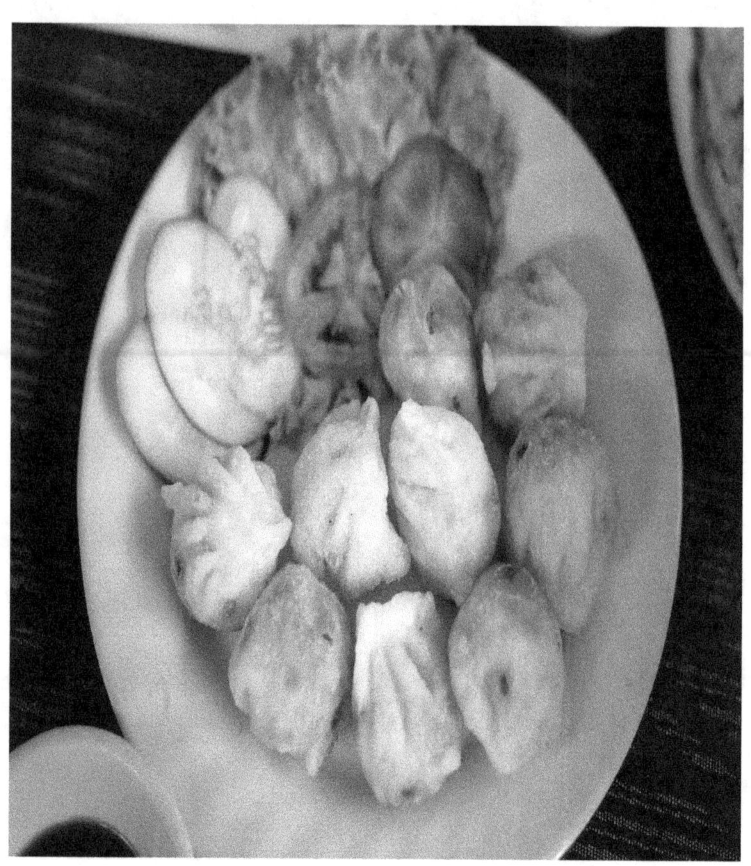

CHAPTER 4

LOW FOODMAP FOODS

Low FODMAP foods are those with lower levels of specific carbohydrates that can ferment in the gut, causing symptoms like bloating, gas, and abdominal pain. Examples of low FODMAP foods include:

1. Fruits: Strawberries, blueberries, grapes, oranges, and bananas.
2. Vegetables: Carrots, zucchini, cucumbers, lettuce, and bell peppers.
3. Proteins: Most meats, fish, eggs, and tofu.
4. Grains: Rice, oats, quinoa, and gluten-free products.
5. Dairy: Lactose-free milk, hard cheeses, and lactose-free yogurt.
6. Nuts and Seeds: Almonds (in moderation), sunflower seeds, and pumpkin seeds.

It's important to note that a low FODMAP diet is typically followed in three phases: restriction, reintroduction, and maintenance.

COMPREHENSIVE LIST OF LOW FOODMAP FOODS.

Creating a comprehensive list of low FODMAP foods is quite extensive, here's a brief overview by category:

1. Vegetables:
   - Carrots
   - Bell peppers
   - Zucchini
   - Cucumbers
   - Spinach

2. Fruits:
   - Strawberries
   - Blueberries
   - Grapes
   - Kiwi
   - Oranges
3. Proteins:
   - Chicken
   - Turkey
   - Fish (e.g., salmon, cod)
   - Tofu
   - Eggs
4. Grains:
   - Rice
   - Quinoa
   - Oats (limited)
   - Polenta
   - Buckwheat
5. Dairy:
   - Lactose-free milk
   - Hard cheeses (e.g., cheddar, Swiss)
   - lactose-free yogurt
6. Nuts and seeds:
   - Almonds (limited)
   - Walnuts
   - Chia seeds
   - Sunflower seeds
7. Fats and Oils:
   - Olive oil
   - Coconut oil
   - Butter (lactose-free)
8. Beverages:
   - Water
   - Herbal teas
   - Coffee (in moderation)
   - Almond milk (low FODMAP varieties)

RECIPES IDEAS AND MEAL SUGGESTIONS

Certainly! Let's start with a few recipes and meal suggestions that focus on low FODMAP options:

1. Grilled Chicken Salad:
   - Marinate chicken in olive oil, garlic-infused oil, and herbs.
   - Grill until fully cooked and slice into strips.
   - Toss with mixed greens, cherry tomatoes, cucumber, and a light lemon vinaigrette.
2. Quinoa Stir-Fry:
   - Cook quinoa separately.
   - Stir-fry bell peppers, zucchini, and carrots in a low FODMAP stir-fry sauce.
   - Combine with quinoa and add grilled shrimp or tofu for protein.
3. Low FODMAP Zucchini Noodles with Pesto:
   - Spiralize zucchini into noodles.
   - Mix with homemade basil pesto (basil, pine nuts, Parmesan, and garlic-infused oil).
   - Top with grilled cherry tomatoes and grilled chicken.
4. Salmon and Asparagus Parcels:
   - Use parchment paper to wrap the asparagus and salmon fillets.
   - Season with dill, lemon, and a touch of olive oil.
   - Bake the asparagus and salmon together until they are soft and flaky.
5. Turkey and Spinach Stuffed Peppers:
   - Cook ground turkey with low FODMAP spices.
   - Mix with sautéed spinach.
   - Stuff bell peppers and bake until peppers are soft.

Meal Suggestions:

- Breakfast:
   a. Scrambled eggs with spinach and cherry tomatoes.
   b. Served with a side of lactose-free yogurt.
- Lunch:
   a. Quinoa salad with cucumber, red pepper, and feta.

- b. Grilled chicken or tofu for added protein.
- Dinner:
    - a. Grilled fish with a side of roasted sweet potatoes and green beans.
    - b. Add a drizzle of olive oil and a pinch of chives.

Modify these recipes to suit your taste and dietary preferences. Change portion sizes to meet your nutritional needs and savor a range of delicious low FODMAP meals!

TIPS FOR NAVIGATING RESTAURANTS AND SOCIAL SITUATIONS

- Plan ahead: Check the menu online before you go to the restaurant and look for dishes that are low in FODMAPs or can be easily modified. You can also call the restaurant in advance and ask about the ingredients and preparation methods of the dishes you are interested in. If possible, choose a restaurant that has a variety of gluten-free options, as these are often lower in FODMAPs than wheat-based dishes.
- Communicate your needs: When ordering, politely inform your server of your dietary restrictions and ask for any adjustments or substitutions that can make your meal low FODMAP. For example, you can ask for sauces or dressings to be served on the side, or for onion and garlic to be omitted from your dish. You can also bring your own low FODMAP condiments or snacks to add flavor and variety to your meal.
- Choose wisely: Some cuisines are more low FODMAP-friendly than others. For example, Asian cuisines tend to use a lot of onion, garlic, and soy sauce, which are high in FODMAPs. On the other hand, Mediterranean or Mexican cuisines can offer more low FODMAP options, such as rice, corn tortillas, cheese, meat, fish, and low FODMAP vegetables. You can also opt for simple dishes, such as grilled or roasted meat or fish with a side of salad or steamed vegetables, or gluten-free pasta with olive oil and low FODMAP cheese.
- Enjoy in moderation: Even if you follow the low FODMAP diet, you may still experience some symptoms if you eat too much or too fast. Therefore, it is important to eat slowly, chew well, and pay attention to your hunger and fullness

cues. You can also limit your intake of alcohol, caffeine, and spicy foods, as these can irritate your gut and worsen your symptoms.

- Be flexible and positive: Eating out on the low FODMAP diet can be stressful and frustrating, but it does not have to be. Remember that the diet is not meant to be followed strictly forever, but rather as a temporary tool to identify your triggers and improve your symptoms. You can still enjoy eating out and socializing with your loved ones, as long as you make informed choices and focus on the positive aspects of the experience.

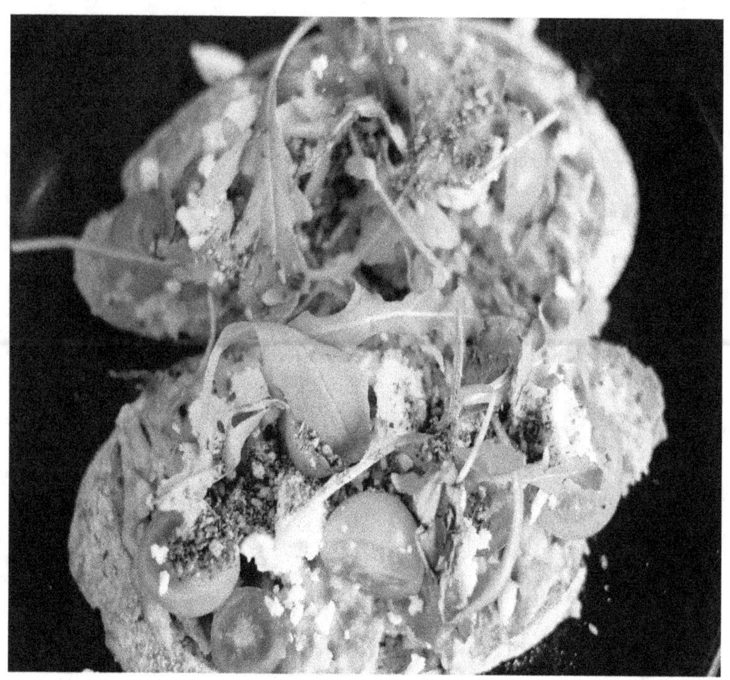

CHAPTER 5

HIGH FOODMAP FOODS TO AVOID

High FODMAP foods that may trigger digestive issues like bloating and discomfort in sensitive individuals. Examples include onions, garlic, certain fruits, and wheat. Avoiding these foods helps manage symptoms in those with irritable bowel syndrome (IBS) or other gastrointestinal conditions sensitive to FODMAPs.

DETAILED LIST OF HIGH FODMAP FOODS TO AVOID

High FODMAP foods to avoid include:

1. Fructose:
   - Honey
   - Agave nectar
   - High fructose corn syrup
   - Some fruits like apples, pears, and watermelon
2. Lactose:
   - Milk (cow, goat, or sheep)
   - Yogurt
   - Soft cheeses (e.g., ricotta, cottage cheese)
3. Fructans:
   - Wheat-based products (bread, pasta)
   - Onion
   - Garlic
   - Inulin-containing foods (chicory root, certain prebiotics)
4. Galactans:
   - Legumes (beans, lentils, chickpeas)
   - Certain vegetables like broccoli, cabbage, and Brussels sprouts
5. Polyols:
   - Stone fruits (e.g., cherries, peaches, plums)
   - Artificial sweeteners with sorbitol, mannitol, xylitol

COMMON PITFALLS AND HIDDEN SOURCES OF FODMAP.

Certainly! Here are some common pitfalls and hidden sources of FODMAPs (Fermentable Oligosaccharides, Disaccharides, Monosaccharides, and Polyols) that individuals with irritable bowel syndrome (IBS) should be aware of:

1. Misunderstanding Portion Sizes:
   a. Pitfall: Consuming large portions of low-FODMAP foods can still lead to high FODMAP intake.
   b. Explanation: It's crucial to be mindful of portion sizes, as even low-FODMAP foods can contribute to symptoms if consumed in excessive amounts.
2. Hidden High-FODMAP Ingredients:
   a. Pitfall: Overlooking ingredients containing high FODMAPs in processed foods.
   b. Explanation: Some packaged foods may contain hidden high-FODMAP ingredients like onion or garlic powder, high-fructose corn syrup, or certain sweeteners. Reading labels is essential.
3. Undetected Polyol Sources:
   a. Pitfall: Missing sources of polyols in seemingly innocent foods.
   b. Explanation: Foods like stone fruits (e.g., cherries, peaches), artificial sweeteners (sorbitol, mannitol), and certain vegetables (e.g., cauliflower) can be high in polyols, contributing to symptoms if not accounted for.
4. Lactose Miscalculations:
   a. Pitfall: Underestimating lactose content in dairy products.
   b. Explanation: Even some lactose-free products may contain trace amounts of lactose. It's important to check labels and opt for lactose-free alternatives if lactose is a trigger.
5. High-FODMAP Health Foods:
   a. Pitfall: Assuming all health foods are low in FODMAPs.
   b. Explanation: Some nutritious foods, such as avocados, honey, or certain legumes, can be high in FODMAPs. Balancing nutritional needs while adhering to a low-FODMAP diet requires careful selection.
6. Condiment Concerns:
   a. Pitfall: Overlooking high-FODMAP ingredients in condiments.

      b. Explanation: Sauces and condiments often contain garlic or onion. Opting for homemade or FODMAP-friendly alternatives is crucial to avoid unnecessary triggers.

7. Cross-Contamination Risks:
   a. Pitfall: Neglecting cross-contamination in food preparation.
   b. Explanation: Shared cooking utensils or surfaces used for high-FODMAP and low-FODMAP foods can lead to unintentional contamination. Maintaining a separate preparation area is key.

8. Unrecognized Fructan Sources:
   a. Pitfall: Ignoring sources of hidden fructans.
   b. Explanation: Foods like wheat, rye, and barley are high in fructans. Checking ingredient lists for wheat-based additives in processed foods is vital for avoiding unnecessary fructan intake.

9. Inadequate Food Diary:
   a. Pitfall: Not keeping an accurate food diary.
   b. Explanation: Without a detailed food diary, it can be challenging to identify specific trigger foods and patterns. A well-maintained diary helps in pinpointing sources of discomfort.

10. Ignoring Personal Tolerance Levels:
    a. Pitfall: Assuming universal tolerance levels for all low-FODMAP foods.
    b. Explanation: Individual tolerance varies. Some may tolerate certain moderate-FODMAP foods, while others may not. It's essential to tailor the diet based on personal response.

Understanding and navigating these common pitfalls can enhance the effectiveness of a low-FODMAP diet in managing IBS symptoms. For individualized guidance, always speak with a medical professional or registered dietitian.

LABEL READING AND INGREDIENT AWARENESS

Label reading and ingredient awareness are crucial aspects, especially for individuals following a low FODMAP diet. When reading labels on food products for a low FODMAP diet, focus on identifying specific ingredients that may trigger digestive discomfort. High-FODMAP ingredients to watch out for include fructose, lactose, fructans, galactans, and polyols. You can make better decisions if you are familiar with these terminology..

Check for hidden sources of FODMAPs. Ingredients like wheat, onions, garlic, and certain sweeteners may contain FODMAPs. Manufacturers often use alternative names for these ingredients, so being vigilant is essential. Look for terms like inulin, chicory root extract, and high fructose corn syrup, as they may indicate the presence of FODMAPs.

Understanding serving sizes is critical. A product may be low FODMAP in small quantities but become high FODMAP in larger portions. Pay attention to the recommended serving sizes provided on labels to ensure you stay within the safe limits.

Opt for products with clear labeling. Some food manufacturers now include low FODMAP labels, making it easier for individuals to identify suitable products quickly. Look for certifications or statements on the packaging that indicate the product is FODMAP-friendly.

Utilize smartphone apps and resources. There are apps designed to assist individuals following a low FODMAP diet by providing information about specific products and ingredients. These tools can be valuable companions when navigating the grocery store aisles.

In summary, label reading and ingredient awareness are vital components of successfully managing a low FODMAP diet. By familiarizing yourself with high-FODMAP ingredients, checking for hidden sources, understanding serving sizes, and utilizing available resources, you can make informed choices to support your digestive health.

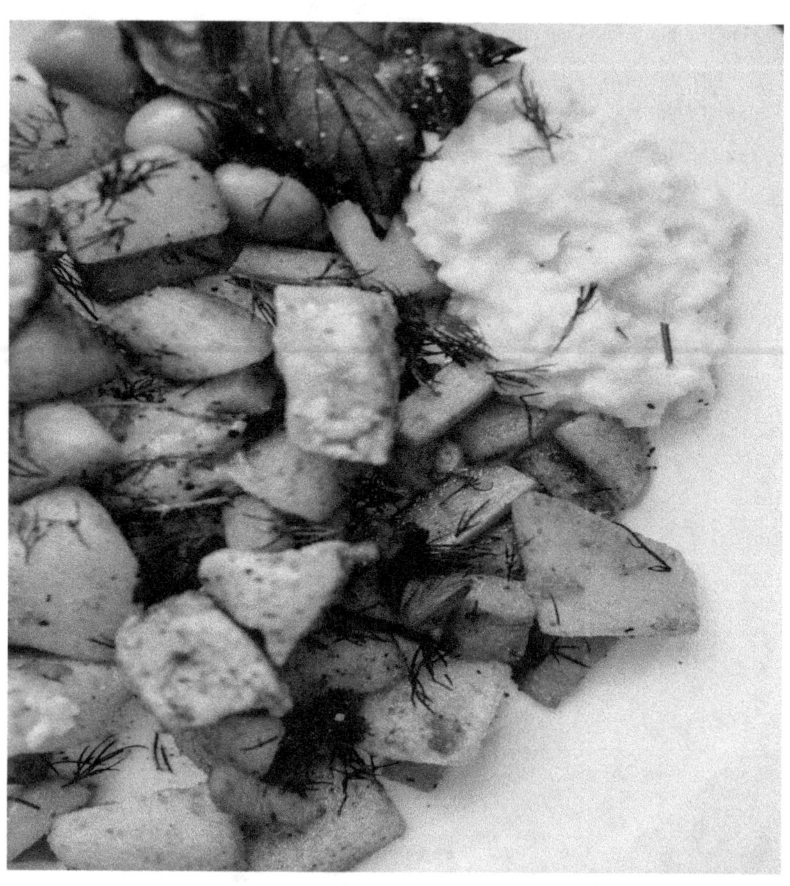

CHAPTER 6

MEAL PLANNING AND RECIPES

Meal planning is setting up and cooking meals ahead of time, usually for a week. It helps save time, money, and ensures a balanced diet. Recipes are detailed instructions for preparing specific dishes, providing a step-by-step guide on ingredients and cooking methods. Together, meal planning and recipes streamline the cooking process and contribute to healthier eating habits.

SAMPLE MEAL PLANS FOR DIFFERENT DIETARY PREFERENCES.

Here are sample FODMAP-friendly meal plans for various dietary preferences:

1. Vegetarian FODMAP Meal Plan:

Breakfast: Quinoa porridge with lactose-free milk, topped with strawberries.
Lunch: Grilled tofu and vegetable stir-fry with rice.
Dinner: Lentil soup with green beans and a side of baked sweet potatoes.

2. Low FODMAP Paleo Meal Plan:

Breakfast: Scrambled eggs with spinach and grilled tomatoes.
Lunch: Grilled chicken salad with mixed greens, carrots, and a simple olive oil dressing.
Dinner: Baked salmon with roasted zucchini and mashed parsnips.

3. Gluten-Free FODMAP Meal Plan:

Breakfast: Omelette with bacon, tomatoes, and lactose-free cheese.
Lunch: Quinoa salad with cucumber, bell peppers, and grilled chicken.
Dinner: Gluten-free pasta with a homemade tomato and basil sauce, topped with

ground turkey.

4. **Vegan FODMAP Meal Plan:**

Breakfast: Chia seed pudding made with almond milk, topped with blueberries.
Lunch: Chickpea and spinach curry with basmati rice.
Dinner: Grilled eggplant and zucchini stacks with a tomato and herbs sauce.

5. **Low FODMAP Mediterranean Meal Plan:**

Breakfast: Greek yogurt with strawberries and a sprinkle of pumpkin seeds.
Lunch: Mediterranean quinoa salad with olives, cherry tomatoes, and feta cheese.
Dinner: Grilled shrimp with lemon, oregano, and a side of roasted bell peppers.

6. **Keto FODMAP Meal Plan:**

Breakfast: Avocado and bacon egg cups.
Lunch consists of grilled chicken and zucchini noodles with pesto.
Dinner: Steak with a side of sautéed spinach and buttered green beans.

LOW FODMAP SAMPLE MEAL PLANS FOR DIFFERENT DIETARY PREFERENCES

Now diving in into the real low FODMAP sample meal plans for various dietary preferences which includes:

1. **Low FODMAP Vegetarian Meal Plan:**

- Breakfast: Scrambled eggs with spinach and tomatoes.
- Lunch: Quinoa salad with cucumber, bell peppers, and feta cheese.
- Dinner: Grilled tofu with steamed broccoli and carrots.
- Snacks: Almonds and lactose-free yogurt.

2. Low FODMAP Paleo Meal Plan:

- Breakfast: Omelette with bacon, spinach, and mushrooms.
- Lunch: Grilled chicken breast with mixed greens and olive oil.
- Dinner: Baked salmon with roasted sweet potatoes and asparagus.
- Snacks: Carrot sticks with almond butter.

3. Low FODMAP Mediterranean Meal Plan:

- Breakfast: Greek yogurt with strawberries and a sprinkle of chia seeds.
- Lunch: Mediterranean salad with olives, cherry tomatoes, and grilled chicken.
- Dinner: Baked cod with lemon, capers, and a side of quinoa.
- Snacks: Hummus with cucumber slices.

4. Low FODMAP Vegan Meal Plan:

- Breakfast: Smoothie with banana (underripe), spinach, and almond milk.
- Lunch: Lentil soup with carrots, zucchini, and a side of mixed greens.
- Dinner: Stir-fried tempeh with bok choy and bell peppers.
- Snacks: Rice cakes with peanut butter.

5. Low FODMAP Gluten-Free Meal Plan:

- Breakfast: Gluten-free oats with strawberries and lactose-free milk.
- Lunch: Quinoa and grilled chicken bowl with tomatoes and cucumbers.
- Dinner: Shrimp stir-fry with broccoli, bell peppers, and gluten-free soy sauce.
- Snacks: Rice crackers with cheddar cheese.

EASY AND DELICIOUS LOW FOODMAP RECIPES

Low FODMAP recipes are suitable for people who have digestive issues such as irritable bowel syndrome (IBS). They avoid foods that contain high amounts of fermentable carbohydrates, which can trigger symptoms like bloating, gas, and pain. Here are some easy and delicious low FODMAP recipes with detailed explanations:

- Lemon-Butter Tilapia with Almonds: This is a simple and quick fish dish that is low in FODMAPs and high in protein and healthy fats. You just need tilapia fillets, butter, lemon juice, parsley, salt, pepper, and sliced almonds. You can bake the fish in the oven or cook it in a skillet, then top it with the buttery lemon sauce and almonds. Serve it with a green salad or steamed vegetables for a complete meal.

- Lemon Cranberry Quinoa Salad: This is a refreshing and nutritious salad that is perfect for lunch or as a side dish. You need cooked quinoa, dried cranberries, chopped parsley, lemon juice, olive oil, salt, and pepper. You can also add some chopped walnuts or pecans for extra crunch and flavor. Toss everything together in a large bowl and enjoy cold or at room temperature.

- Egg Drop Soup: This is a classic Chinese soup that is low in FODMAPs and very easy to make. You need chicken broth, soy sauce, sesame oil, cornstarch, water, eggs, and green onion tops. You can also add some shredded chicken, tofu, or cooked rice for more substance. You just need to bring the broth to a boil, then whisk in the cornstarch mixture to thicken it. Then, slowly drizzle in the beaten eggs while stirring the soup to create thin ribbons. Garnish with green onion tops and serve hot.

- [Broiled Cod]: This is another simple and tasty fish recipe that is low in FODMAPs and high in omega-3 fatty acids. You need cod fillets, olive oil, lemon juice, garlic-infused oil, salt, pepper, and parsley. You can broil the fish in the oven or grill it on a barbecue, then drizzle it with the garlic-lemon sauce and sprinkle with parsley. Serve it with roasted potatoes or rice and a low FODMAP vegetable of your choice.

- [Cranberry-Walnut Oatmeal]: This is a warm and cozy breakfast that is low in FODMAPs and high in fiber and antioxidants. You need rolled oats, water, milk, salt, brown sugar, cinnamon, dried cranberries, and chopped walnuts. You can cook the oatmeal on the stovetop or in the microwave, then stir in the brown sugar, cinnamon, cranberries, and walnuts. You can also add some maple syrup, vanilla extract, or nut butter for more flavor and sweetness.

These are just some examples of low FODMAP recipes that you can try. That can help you manage your digestive issues while enjoying a variety of foods. You can find more low FODMAP recipes on the websites FODMAP Everyday and Monash Fodmap.

COOKING TIPS AND TRICKS.

Certainly! Here are some cooking tips and tricks for a low FODMAP diet:

1. Choose FODMAP-friendly ingredients:
   - Opt for low FODMAP alternatives like green leafy vegetables, carrots, zucchini, and gluten-free grains such as quinoa or rice.
2. Mindful seasoning:
   - Use herbs and spices like garlic-infused oil, chives, and oregano for flavor without excess FODMAPs.
3. Experiment with lactose-free dairy:
   - Incorporate lactose-free options like lactose-free milk or hard cheeses to avoid high FODMAP levels in regular dairy.
4. Watch portion sizes:
   - Keep servings of moderate FODMAP foods in check to prevent exceeding individual tolerance levels.
5. Homemade stock and broth:

- o Make your own broths using low FODMAP vegetables and herbs to control the ingredients and flavors.
6. Select gluten-free grains:
   - o Embrace grains like quinoa, rice, and oats without gluten to reduce FODMAP intake.
7. Mindful fruit choices:
   - o Opt for low FODMAP fruits like berries, kiwi, and citrus, and be cautious with high FODMAP options like apples and stone fruits.
8. Limit onion and garlic:
   - o Use infused oils, chives, or green parts of spring onions to impart flavor without the high FODMAP content found in onion and garlic.
9. Experiment with alternative sweeteners:
   - o Try sweeteners like maple syrup, golden syrup, or stevia instead of honey or high FODMAP sweeteners.
10. Prevent cross-contamination:
   - o Clean cooking utensils and surfaces thoroughly to avoid mixing high and low FODMAP ingredients.
11. Opt for homemade sauces and dressings:
   - o Create your own sauces and dressings to control ingredients, avoiding excess FODMAPs found in some store-bought options.
12. Be mindful of hidden FODMAPs:
   - o Check labels for hidden sources of FODMAPs in packaged foods, such as onion powder or high-fructose corn syrup.
13. Experiment with alternative flours:
   - o Use gluten-free flours like rice flour or almond flour in baking to reduce FODMAPs.
14. Slow-cooking and marinating:
   - o Marinate proteins with low FODMAP ingredients and opt for slow-cooking methods to enhance flavors without relying on high FODMAP ingredients.
15. Stay hydrated:
   - o Drink plenty of water and herbal teas to support digestion and overall well-being.

CHAPTER 7

OVERCOMING CHALLENGES

Overcoming challenges with the FODMAP diet involves persistence and gradual adjustments. Initially daunting, understanding trigger foods and experimenting with alternatives is key. Building a supportive routine and seeking guidance from healthcare professionals make the journey more manageable. It's a process of self-discovery and adapting to a new way of eating, but the positive impact on digestive health Is worth the effort.

DEALING WITH CRAVINGS AND FOOD RESTRICTIONS.

Dealing with cravings and adhering to food restrictions can be a challenging yet essential aspect of maintaining a healthy lifestyle. Whether you're following a specific diet plan, managing allergies, or pursuing weight loss goals, understanding how to handle cravings and navigate food restrictions is crucial for long-term success.

Understanding Cravings:

1. Physical, psychological, and environmental variables frequently interact to cause cravings. Recognizing the triggers behind cravings is the first step in effectively managing them. Common causes include emotional stress, hormonal fluctuations, and exposure to tempting food cues.

Mindful Eating:

2. Practicing mindful eating involves being fully present during meals, paying attention to hunger and fullness cues, and savoring each bite. This approach helps foster a deeper connection with food, making it easier to identify true hunger and distinguish it from cravings.

Meal Planning and Preparation:

3. Strategically planning and preparing meals in advance can help curb cravings by ensuring that nutritious options are readily available. Include a balance of macronutrients and incorporate a variety of flavors to make your meals satisfying and enjoyable.

Substitution and Healthy Alternatives:

4. Instead of succumbing to unhealthy cravings, explore nutritious alternatives that align with your dietary restrictions. For example, if craving something sweet, opt for fruits or naturally sweetened snacks. This allows you to satisfy your cravings while maintaining a healthy eating pattern.

Hydration and Nutrient Intake:

5. Adequate hydration is often overlooked but plays a vital role in managing cravings. Sometimes the body misinterprets thirst for hunger.Ensure you're well-hydrated throughout the day, and prioritize nutrient-dense foods to meet your body's nutritional needs.

Emotional Regulation:

6. Cravings are closely tied to emotions, and addressing emotional well-being is crucial. Engage in stress-reducing activities such as meditation, exercise, or hobbies to manage emotions without resorting to unhealthy food choices.

Seeking Professional Guidance:

7. If dealing with specific dietary restrictions or health conditions, consulting with a registered dietitian or healthcare professional can provide personalized guidance. They can help create a tailored nutrition plan that aligns with your goals while accommodating any limitations.

Building a Support System:

8. With family, friends, or a support group, tell them about your adventure.Having a network of individuals who understand your goals and challenges can provide encouragement and accountability, making it easier to stay on track.

Effectively managing cravings and navigating food restrictions is a dynamic process that requires a combination of self-awareness, planning, and resilience. By understanding the root causes of cravings, adopting mindful eating practices, and incorporating healthy alternatives, individuals can foster a positive relationship with food while maintaining dietary goals.

COMMON ISSUES ON THE LOW FODMAP DIET

Some people, especially those with irritable bowel syndrome (IBS) or small intestinal bacterial overgrowth (SIBO), may have difficulty digesting and absorbing FODMAPs. This can lead to increased water and gas in the intestine, which can trigger or worsen the symptoms mentioned above. By following a low FODMAP diet, these people may experience significant improvement in their digestive health and quality of life.

However, the low FODMAP diet is not without challenges and limitations. Some of the common issues that may arise from following this diet are:

- It is a restrictive and complex diet that requires careful planning and guidance from a qualified health professional, such as a doctor or a dietitian. There are three stages to the diet: personalization, reintroduction, and elimination.In the elimination phase, all high FODMAP foods are avoided for two to six weeks. In the reintroduction phase, each FODMAP group is tested one by one to identify the individual tolerance and trigger foods. In the personalization phase, a long-term diet is established based on the results of the reintroduction phase. This process can be time-consuming, challenging, and confusing for some people.
- It is not a one-size-fits-all diet that works for everyone. The response to the low FODMAP diet may vary depending on the individual's underlying condition, symptoms, FODMAP tolerance, and dietary preferences. Some people may see significant improvement, while others may see little or no change. Some people may also have other factors that contribute to their digestive symptoms, such as stress, anxiety, medications, or other food intolerances. Therefore, the low FODMAP diet should not be considered as the only or the ultimate solution for digestive problems.
- It is not a permanent or a long-term diet that can be followed indefinitely. The low FODMAP diet is meant to be a temporary and a short-term intervention that helps identify and avoid the problematic foods for each person. Staying on a low FODMAP diet for too long can have negative consequences, such as nutritional deficiencies, reduced gut microbiota diversity, increased risk of chronic diseases, and reduced social and emotional well-being. Therefore, it is important to reintroduce and include as many high FODMAP foods as tolerated in the diet, and to seek professional advice on how to balance the diet with adequate nutrition and variety.

The low FODMAP diet can be a useful and effective tool for managing digestive symptoms in some people, but it is not without drawbacks and challenges. It is essential to consult with a health professional before starting the diet, and to follow the diet instructions carefully and correctly. The low FODMAP diet should also be seen as a part of a holistic approach that addresses the physical, mental, and emotional aspects of digestive health.

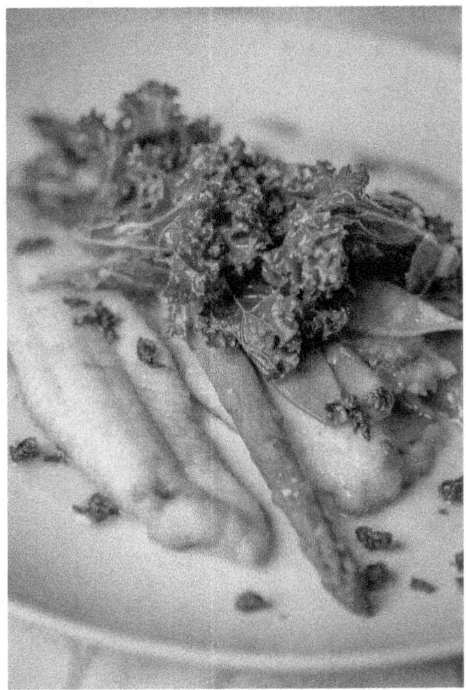

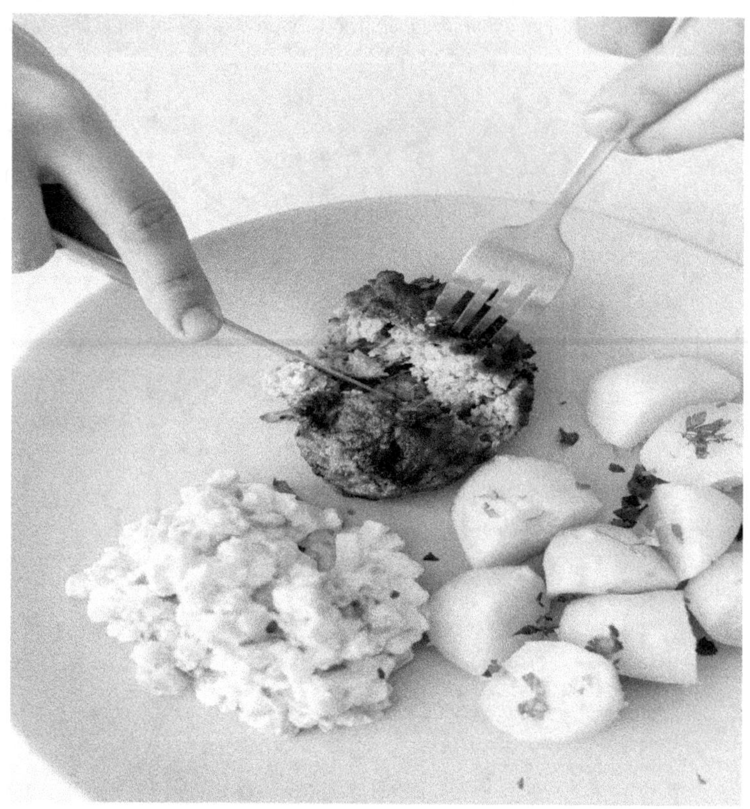

CHAPTER 8

MONITORING AND REINTRODUCTION

"Eat to beat your diet" involves a strategic approach to food consumption, emphasizing monitoring, reintroduction, and personalized adjustments.

Monitoring Symptoms:

Careful observation of how your body responds to different foods is crucial. Note digestive symptoms, energy levels, and overall well-being. This self-awareness forms the foundation for understanding your body's unique reactions.

Reintroducing FODMAPs:

FODMAPs are fermentable carbohydrates that some individuals find challenging to digest. Gradually reintroduce specific FODMAP-containing foods, monitoring your body's response. This systematic reintroduction helps identify trigger foods and allows for a more nuanced understanding of individual tolerances.

Adjusting the Diet Based on Individual Responses:

Every individual's body is distinct. Analyze the collected data from monitoring symptoms and FODMAP reintroduction. Adjust your diet accordingly, focusing on what suits your body best. This iterative process enables a personalized and sustainable approach to nutrition.

In essence, "eating to beat your diet" involves a dynamic and informed relationship with food, where observation and adaptation play key roles in achieving a diet that aligns with your unique physiological needs.

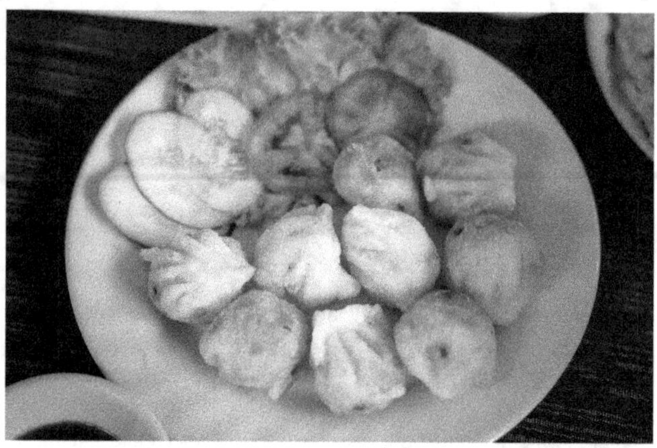

CHAPTER 8

LONG-TERM MAINTENANCE

The low FODMAP diet is a dietary approach that aims to reduce the intake of high FODMAP foods and identify the individual triggers and tolerances of each person. It consists of three phases: elimination, reintroduction and personalization.

The elimination phase involves following a strict low FODMAP diet for 2 to 6 weeks, or until significant symptom improvement is achieved. This phase helps to calm down the gut and establish a baseline for further testing.

The reintroduction phase involves systematically testing each FODMAP group in a controlled manner, using specific foods and serving sizes. This phase helps to determine which FODMAPs cause symptoms and at what level of intake. .

The personalization phase involves establishing a long term, personalized FODMAP diet that balances symptom control and nutritional adequacy. This phase involves gradually increasing the intake of well-tolerated FODMAPs and avoiding only the foods that trigger symptoms. The goal is to follow the least restrictive diet possible, while maintaining a good quality of life.

Some general tips for maintaining a long term, personalized FODMAP diet are:

- Adhere to a regular meal pattern and avoid skipping meals
- Drink at least 8 cups of fluid per day, especially water or non-caffeinated drinks
- Reduce your consumption of tea, coffee, carbonated drinks, and alcohol.
- Eat fewer foods high in insoluble fiber, such as bran.)
- Include a variety of low FODMAP foods from all food groups
- Use the Monash FODMAP app or other reliable sources to check the FODMAP content of foods and serving sizes
- Read food labels carefully and look for hidden FODMAPs in ingredients and additives
- Experiment with different herbs, spices and condiments to add flavor and variety to your meals
- Plan ahead and prepare low FODMAP snacks and meals for when you are out or traveling
- Seek professional advice from a registered dietitian if you have any concerns or questions about your diet

CONCLUSION

In conclusion, embracing a low FODMAP diet as a beginner involves key principles. First, familiarize yourself with low FODMAP foods to manage digestive symptoms effectively. Remember to gradually reintroduce higher FODMAP foods to identify personal triggers. Prioritize balanced nutrition by including a variety of tolerated foods in your diet.

For ongoing support and education, consider exploring reputable resources. Websites like Monash University's FODMAP app provide valuable information, and registered dietitians can offer personalized guidance. Connecting with online communities, such as forums or social media groups, allows you to share experiences and gain insights from others on a similar journey.

Embrace this dietary approach with patience and optimism, as understanding your body's response to FODMAPs is a gradual process. With diligence and support, you can navigate the low FODMAP lifestyle successfully, promoting better digestive health and overall well-being.